OOPS! IT'S A PACEMAKER!

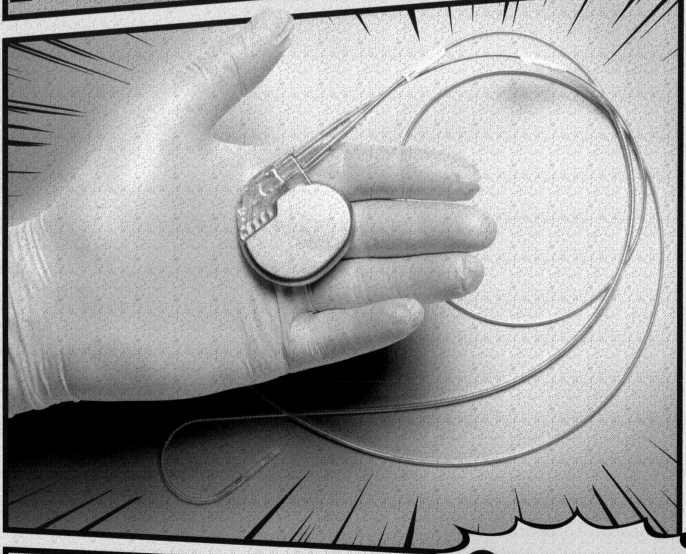

BY JONATHAN BARD

 Gareth Stevens
PUBLISHING

Please visit our website, www.garethstevens.com. For a free color catalog of all our high-quality books, call toll free 1-800-542-2595 or fax 1-877-542-2596.

Library of Congress Cataloging-in-Publication Data

Names: Bard, Jonathan, author.
Title: Oops! It's a pacemaker! / Jonathan Bard.
Other titles: It's a pacemaker | It is a pacemaker
Description: New York : Gareth Stevens, [2020] | Series: Accidental
    scientific discoveries | Includes bibliographical references and index.
Identifiers: LCCN 2018043884| ISBN 9781538239827 (pbk.) | ISBN 9781538239841
    (library bound) | ISBN 9781538239834 (6 pack)
Subjects: LCSH: Cardiac pacemakers–Juvenile literature. |
    Arrhythmia–Juvenile literature. | Heart–Diseases–Juvenile literature. |
    Discoveries in science–Juvenile literature.
Classification: LCC RC684.P3 B3625 2020 | DDC 617.4/120592–dc23
LC record available at https://lccn.loc.gov/2018043884

First Edition

Published in 2020 by
Gareth Stevens Publishing
111 East 14th Street, Suite 349
New York, NY 10003

Copyright © 2020 Gareth Stevens Publishing

Designer: Katelyn E. Reynolds
Editor: Monika Davies

Photo credits: Cover, p. 1 Peter Dazeley/Photographer's Choice/Getty Images; cover, pp. 1–32 (burst) jirawat phueksriphan/Shutterstock.com; cover, pp. 1–32 (burst lines) KID_A/Shutterstock.com; p. 5 (main) David Martin/The White House Historical Association/Scewing/Wikipedia.org ; p. 5 (inset) Ted Thai/The LIFE Picture Collection/Getty Images; p. 7 okili77/Shutterstock.com; p. 9 Monkey Business Images/Shutterstock.com; p. 11 ShutterOK/Shutterstock.com; p. 13 PubMed Central (https://www.ncbi.nlm.nih.gov/pmc/articles/PMC3232561/figure/F40/) CC BY-NC-SA 3.0; p. 15 Keystone/Hulton Archive/Getty Images; p. 17 PubMed Central (https://www.ncbi.nlm.nih.gov/pmc/articles/PMC3232561/figure/F78/) © Images in Paediatric Cardiology/CC BY-NC-SA 3.0; p. 19 PubMed Central (https://www.ncbi.nlm.nih.gov/pmc/articles/PMC3232561/figure/F79/) © Images in Paediatric Cardiology/CC BY-NC-SA 3.0; p. 21 (main) Keystone/Getty Images; p. 21 (inset) The Central Intelligence Agency (https://www.flickr.com/people/59094030@N08/)/Slick-o-bot/Wikipedia.org; p. 23 Richman Photo/Shutterstock.com; p. 25 Joe Raedle/Getty Images; p. 27 Jose Luis Calvo/Shutterstock.com.

Printed in the United States of America

CPSIA compliance information: Batch #CS19GS: For further information contact Gareth Stevens, New York, New York at 1-800-542-2595.

CONTENTS

Words in the glossary appear in **bold** type the first time they are used in the text.

ACCIDENTAL DISCOVERIES IN SCIENCE

An inventor is a person who creates something new that's never been made before. In **laboratories** all around the world, inventors tinker away, trying to think up and make new things. For most successful inventions, their creators kept notes, fixed failed experiments, and perfected their inventions over time.

But not every successful invention is a product of such careful planning and testing. Some are actually the result of very fortunate accidents. One such fortunate accident is the creation of a dependable, **implantable** pacemaker—an invention that even today keeps millions of hearts around the world beating correctly.

AWESOME INVENTIONS

SOME OF THE GREATEST INVENTORS CREATED EVERYDAY OBJECTS WE STILL USE TODAY! MARY ANDERSON INVENTED WINDSHIELD WIPERS FOR VEHICLES. BENJAMIN FRANKLIN INVENTED BIFOCAL GLASSES, WHICH ARE GLASSES SPLIT INTO TWO SECTIONS THAT HELP PEOPLE SEE THINGS THAT ARE CLOSE AND THINGS THAT ARE FAR AWAY. AND, NANCY JOHNSON INVENTED THE HAND-OPERATED ICE CREAM MAKER.

Benjamin Franklin, shown here, invented bifocals in 1784.

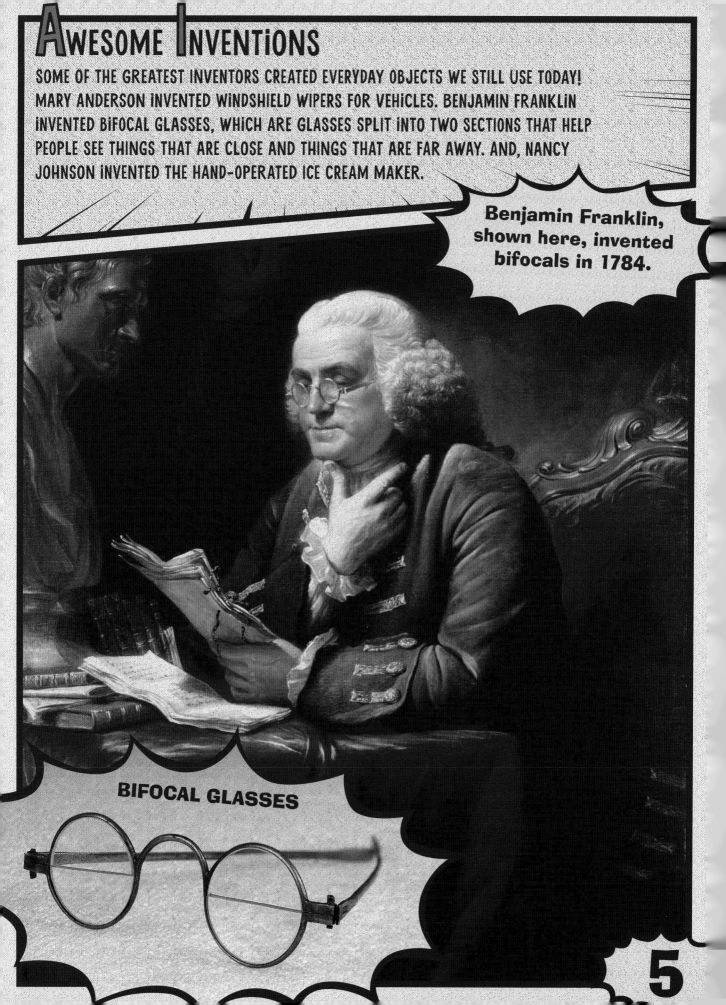

BIFOCAL GLASSES

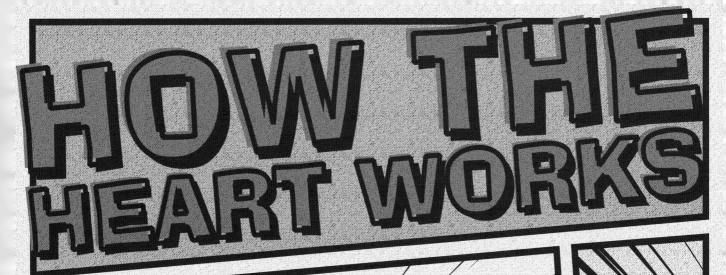

HOW THE HEART WORKS

The heart is the workhorse of our circulatory system. The circulatory system in the human body moves blood to all the **organs**. In the heart, blood flows through four chambers, or areas. Think of the heart as having a left half and a right half, each with two chambers.

The right side of the heart receives oxygen-poor blood from the body. It then pumps this oxygen-poor blood to the lungs. The left side does the opposite, receiving oxygen-rich blood from the lungs, then pumping that blood out to the rest of the body.

YOUR HEART RATE

WHEN YOUR BODY IS AT REST, YOUR HEART TYPICALLY BEATS BETWEEN 60 AND 100 TIMES PER MINUTE. WHEN YOU EXERCISE, YOUR HEART RATE CAN INCREASE UP TO 180 BEATS PER MINUTE! PEOPLE WHO ARE QUITE ATHLETIC AND HEALTHY, SUCH AS OLYMPIC ATHLETES, USUALLY HAVE LOWER HEART RATES.

PARTS
OF THE HEART

Your heart is made of many parts, all of which work together to keep oxygen-rich blood moving around your body to different organs.

AORTA

SUPERIOR VENA CAVA

PULMONARY ARTERY

LEFT ATRIUM

RIGHT ATRIUM

LEFT VENTRICLE

RIGHT VENTRICLE

ELECTRICAL CURRENTS IN THE HEART

For the heart to pump blood through the body, all the parts of the heart must work together. Each chamber has to contract and relax, similar to the action of squeezing and releasing your fist. This pushes blood in and out of the heart. Special cells in the heart known as pacemaker cells send electrical impulses, or signals, to different parts of the heart muscle to tell them when to contract and relax.

These pacemaker cells respond to different situations your body faces. For example, when you exercise, the pacemaker cells speed up your heart rate to pump more blood.

PACEMAKER CELLS

THERE ARE TWO GROUPS OF PACEMAKER CELLS. THE FIRST GROUP MAKES UP THE SINOATRIAL (*SY-NOH-EY-TREE-UHL*) NODE, WHICH STARTS THE ELECTRICAL SIGNAL TO THE HEART MUSCLE. THE SECOND GROUP MAKES UP THE ATRIOVENTRICULAR (*EY-TREE-OH-VEN-TRIK-YUH-LER*) NODE, WHICH SLOWS DOWN THE SIGNAL. TOGETHER, THEY CONTROL HOW FAST THE HEART BEATS AND MAKE SURE THE **VALVES** OPEN AND CLOSE IN THE CORRECT ORDER.

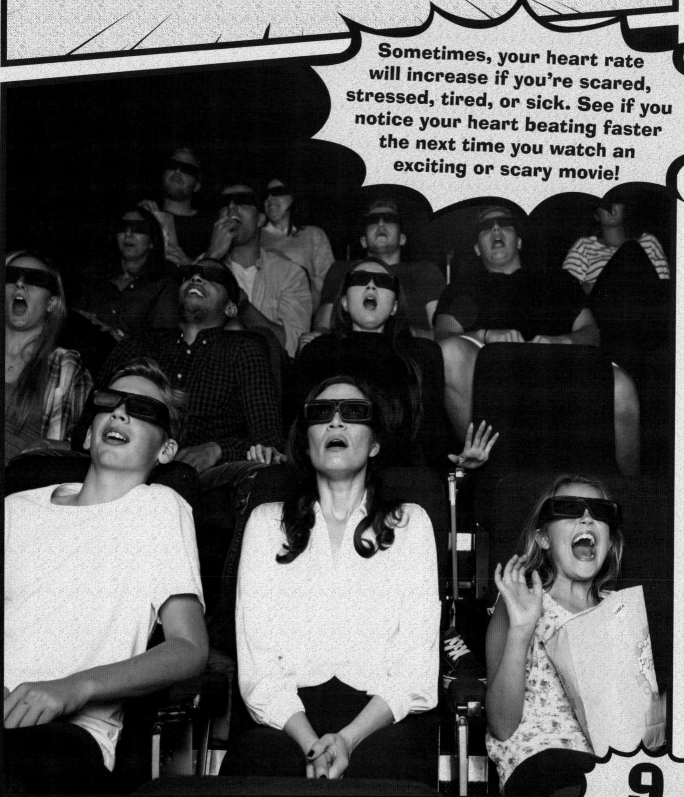

Sometimes, your heart rate will increase if you're scared, stressed, tired, or sick. See if you notice your heart beating faster the next time you watch an exciting or scary movie!

9

WHEN PROBLEMS HAPPEN

Sometimes the heart's timing is off, or it may not beat properly. There are many reasons why someone's heartbeat may become **irregular**. For example, a heart attack may weaken the heart muscle, or an operation may put stress on the heart.

To help treat the problem of an irregular heartbeat, doctors sometimes use artificial pacemakers. Artificial pacemakers are small electronic devices. Unlike the pacemaker cells already inside the heart, artificial pacemakers are mechanical! These devices help the heart beat in time by providing the electric impulses, or signals, that would normally be sent by the heart's pacemaker cells.

ELECTROCARDIOGRAMS

TO CHECK THE ELECTRICAL ACTIVITY OF THE HEART AND RECOGNIZE PROBLEMS, DOCTORS USE A TEST CALLED AN ELECTROCARDIOGRAM, OR ECG. AN ECG SHOWS THE HEARTBEAT AS A BOUNCING LINE ON A SCREEN, AND THERE'S A BEEPING SOUND FOR EVERY BEAT. IN 1905, DUTCH PHYSIOLOGIST DR. WILLEM EINTHOVEN RECORDED THE FIRST HUMAN ELECTROCARDIOGRAM.

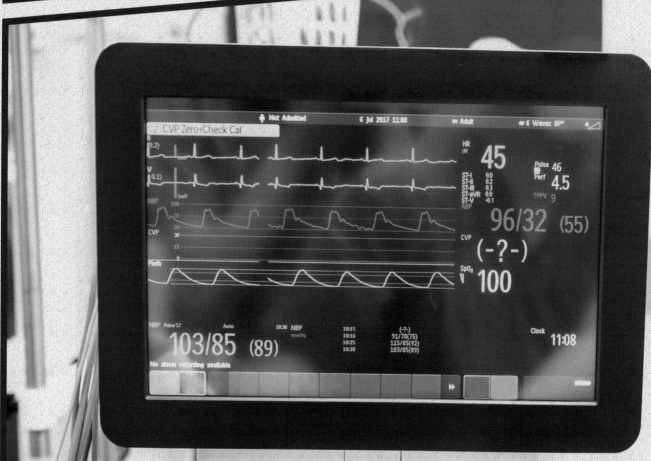

Electrocardiograms are simple and painless tests that can provide a lot of information about how well a person's heart is working.

THE FIRST PACEMAKERS

As early as the 1700s, doctors have been using electricity to help the heart work better. But it wasn't until the 1930s that the first mechanical pacemaker was invented. In 1932, Albert Hyman developed a hand-crank motor that delivered electrical currents through a small needle inserted into the heart.

Over the next 30 years, inventors worked on developing different kinds of pacemakers. Most of these inventions were very large in size. Some were as big as modern microwaves! Many of these first pacemakers also had to be plugged into the wall.

12

INVENTIONS AN OCEAN APART

AROUND THE TIME ALBERT HYMAN WAS WORKING ON HIS ARTIFICIAL PACEMAKER, AUSTRALIAN DOCTOR MARK LIDWILL WAS INVENTING A SIMILAR MACHINE. IN 1928, LIDWILL SUCCESSFULLY USED HIS MACHINE TO SAVE THE LIFE OF A NEWBORN. HYMAN AND LIDWILL MADE THEIR DISCOVERIES AND INVENTIONS COMPLETELY INDEPENDENT FROM EACH OTHER—SEPARATED BY THE PACIFIC OCEAN!

Hyman's pacemaker was not popular at the time because people felt that restarting the heart was unnatural. Fellow scientists ignored his invention.

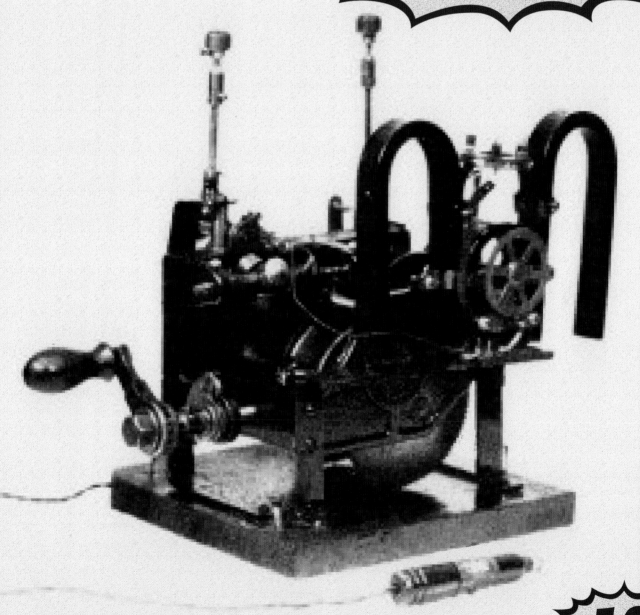

CHALLENGES OF WIDESPREAD USE

Pacemakers still had room for improvement. From the 1930s to the 1960s, medical researchers and inventors tried to make pacemakers smaller and battery powered.

Swedish inventor Rune Elmqvist and Swedish surgeon Åke Senning created the first implantable pacemaker. In the medical world, "implantable" means something placed inside the human body. This was important because it meant people wouldn't have to carry the device with them. Instead, the device would be inside them!

Unfortunately, the first few pacemakers stopped working after only a short time. Inventors needed to find a way for a pacemaker to stay inside the body without needing to be replaced.

The First Human Patient

ARNE LARSSON SUFFERED FROM AN IRREGULAR, SLOW HEARTBEAT, WHICH LED TO STOKES-ADAMS ATTACKS. THESE ATTACKS WOULD CAUSE HIM TO FAINT BECAUSE HIS BLOOD WASN'T PUMPING FAST ENOUGH. HE EXPERIENCED THESE ATTACKS MULTIPLE TIMES A DAY. ARNE LARSSON RECEIVED THE FIRST IMPLANTABLE PACEMAKER FROM ELMQVIST AND SENNING IN 1958. IT ONLY WORKED FOR 8 HOURS.

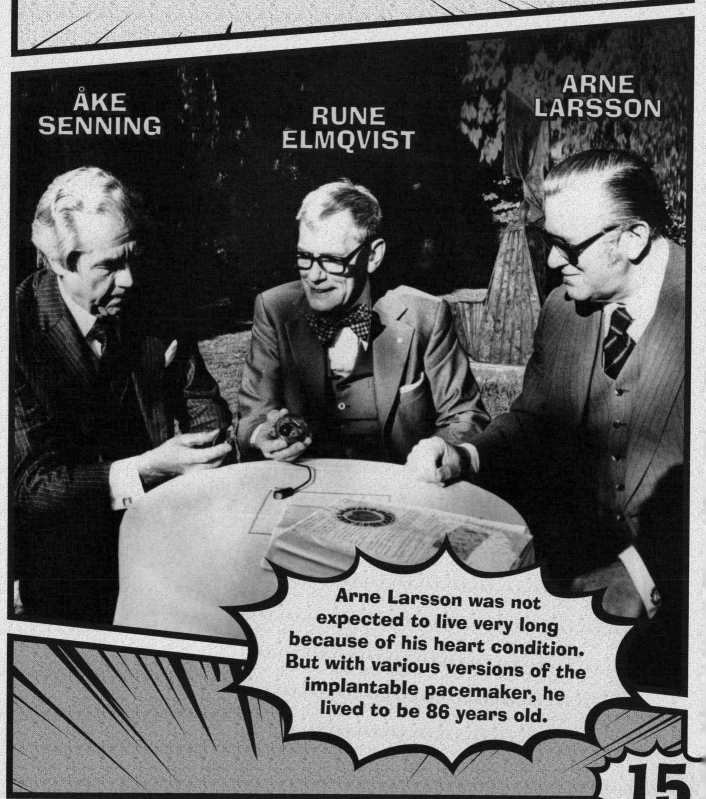

ÅKE SENNING

RUNE ELMQVIST

ARNE LARSSON

Arne Larsson was not expected to live very long because of his heart condition. But with various versions of the implantable pacemaker, he lived to be 86 years old.

OOPS! THE IMPLANTABLE, RELIABLE PACEMAKER

In 1956, American electrical **engineer** Wilson Greatbatch was tinkering with an invention at home. Greatbatch was creating a piece of medical equipment to record heart rates that beat too fast.

While working, he reached into a box to pull out a **resistor**, or a small device that slows down electric current. He accidentally grabbed the wrong one. When he plugged in the wrong resistor, his invention started to buzz in rhythm. Greatbatch immediately realized his invention was buzzing like a heartbeat!

This realization helped Greatbatch create a battery-operated pacemaker that would deliver a pulse or shock to contract the heart muscles. His invention was a big improvement over the pacemakers of the past.

What Is "Squegging"?

WHEN GREATBATCH TURNED ON THE DEVICE THAT WOULD BECOME THE FIRST IMPLANTABLE, RELIABLE PACEMAKER, HE SAID IT STARTED TO "SQUEG." THIS TERM IS USED TO DESCRIBE WHEN AN ELECTRONIC DEVICE BUZZES BRIEFLY AND THEN PAUSES. "SQUEG" COMES FROM THE TERM SELF-QUENCHING. SELF-QUENCHING IS WHEN A DEVICE SWITCHES ITSELF ON AND OFF—LIKE A BEATING HEART!

After his accidental discovery, Greatbatch spent 2 years working in his home laboratory to improve the device. He made over 50 versions of his pacemaker!

GREATBATCH BUILDS A TEAM

After creating multiple versions of his pacemaker and testing them in his laboratory, Greatbatch was ready to test it on a living thing. To do this, he needed a surgeon who believed in his device. Dr. William Chardack, the chief surgeon at a hospital in Buffalo, New York, was his ally in this quest. Assisting Chardack was Dr. Andrew Gage, also a surgeon, and an old friend of Greatbatch.

In 1958, the three men did their first test using an animal's heart. The pacemaker worked, successfully keeping the animal's heart beating in rhythm. This encouraged the team to keep testing, and in 1960, they tested the pacemaker in their first human patient.

The Bow Tie Team

THE THREE MEN BECAME KNOWN AS THE BOW TIE TEAM BECAUSE ALL THREE WORE BOW TIES! THE TWO SURGEONS SAID THEY WORE BOW TIES BECAUSE YOUNG CHILDREN WOULD PULL ON THEIR LONGER NECKTIES. GREATBATCH SAID NECKTIES GOT IN THE WAY WHEN HE WORKED ON HIS INVENTIONS.

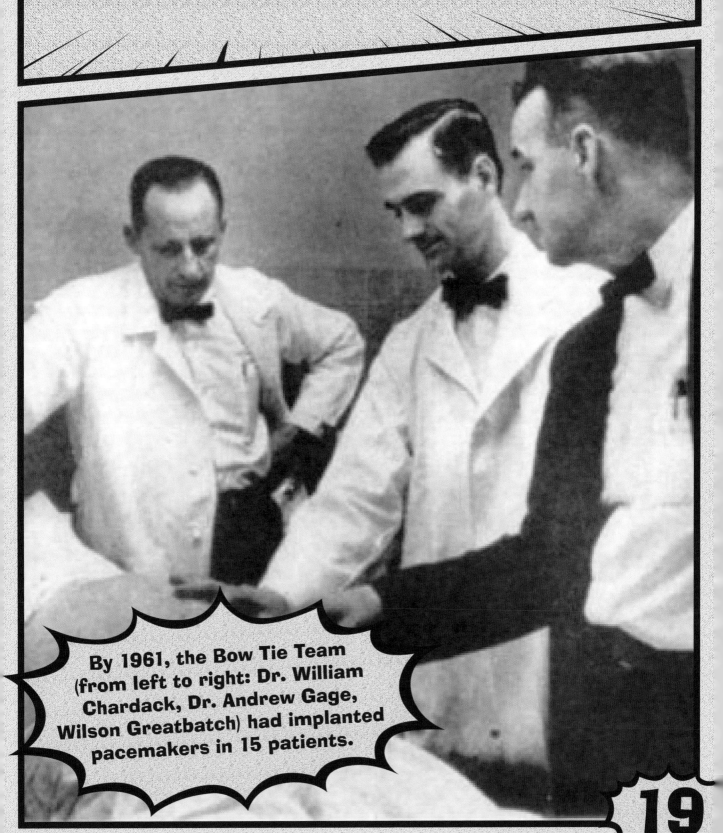

By 1961, the Bow Tie Team (from left to right: Dr. William Chardack, Dr. Andrew Gage, Wilson Greatbatch) had implanted pacemakers in 15 patients.

OVERCOMING PROBLEMS

Once Greatbatch and his team proved his pacemaker worked, they set out to fix the device's problems. The main problem was the batteries. At the time, most pacemaker batteries were zinc-mercury based. But this type of battery had a couple of major problems. First, they didn't last very long. They also **corroded** from being exposed to the inside of the body.

In 1972, Greatbatch and his team invented a new battery using lithium-iodine. This battery could last up to 10 years. The battery was also sealed up, protected from the inside of the body, which prevented corrosion.

Useful Batteries

BATTERIES WORK BY STORING A METAL (SUCH AS LITHIUM) AND A CHEMICAL (SUCH AS IODINE) TOGETHER. THE CHEMICAL TOUCHES THE METAL, CAUSING A CHEMICAL **REACTION** THAT PRODUCES ENERGY. WE USE ENERGY FROM BATTERIES TO POWER MANY THINGS IN OUR LIVES, INCLUDING TOYS, PHONES, VEHICLES, AND MEDICAL DEVICES.

The Central Intelligence Agency (CIA) had been working on lithium-iodine batteries. In the 1960s, the CIA released its research to the public—including Greatbatch—after it had no use for the batteries.

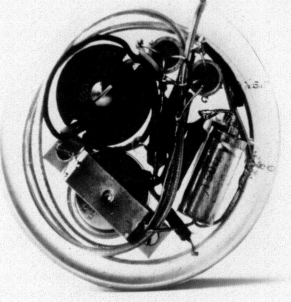

1958 PACEMAKER

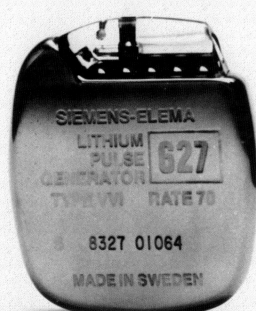

1978 PACEMAKER

CIA'S LITHIUM-IODINE BATTERY

MODERN-DAY PACEMAKERS

Scientists continue to make improvements on the pacemaker. One of the biggest advances is the addition of tiny computers inside pacemakers. These computers record information about the heart's activity. Using this information, they can send signals to the heart to change the heart rate in real time. This helps the pacemaker respond faster to a patient's activities, such as when they're exercising or sleeping.

The internet brought more improvements to the pacemaker. A pacemaker connected to the internet could now send information about the heart's activity directly to doctors. This allowed doctors to watch their patients carefully from afar and spot problems right away.

Internet Connections

THE INTERNET IS A POWERFUL TOOL THAT LETS US SEND AND RECEIVE INFORMATION EASILY. HOWEVER, INTERNET SECURITY IS EXTREMELY IMPORTANT, ESPECIALLY WHEN DEALING WITH MEDICAL DEVICES. THESE DEVICES SEND INFORMATION ABOUT A PATIENT THAT OFTEN CONTAINS PRIVATE DETAILS. THIS IS INFORMATION THAT SHOULD STAY BETWEEN A DOCTOR AND PATIENT AND NOT BE SHARED ON THE INTERNET.

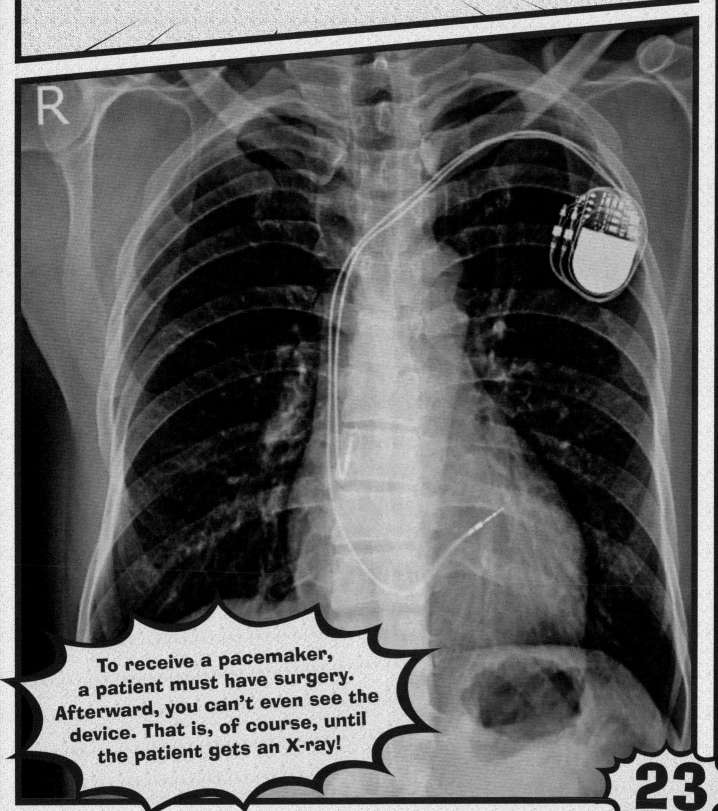

To receive a pacemaker, a patient must have surgery. Afterward, you can't even see the device. That is, of course, until the patient gets an X-ray!

23

LEADLESS PACEMAKERS

Most pacemakers use wires, called leads, to send electrical signals from the pacemaker to the heart. These leads can become a problem if they fall off the heart. Another issue with pacemakers is that the area around the device can become infected, or made ill by bacteria or other disease.

To solve these issues, scientists have removed the leads on a new type of pacemaker. This new pacemaker is placed directly in the heart, which allows it to still deliver the needed electrical signals. This style of pacemaker is called the leadless pacemaker. It doesn't require major surgery, which makes it a lot safer and reduces the risk of getting an infection.

THE FIRST LEADLESS PACEMAKER

IN 2016, THE FIRST LEADLESS PACEMAKER WAS APPROVED FOR USE IN PATIENTS WHO WERE NOT ABLE TO USE TRADITIONAL, OR USUAL, PACEMAKERS. THIS DEVICE IS IMPLANTED INSIDE THE HEART INSTEAD OF BESIDE OR ON THE HEART. IT HAS PROVEN TO BE EFFECTIVE IN OVER 98 PERCENT OF THE PATIENTS WHO RECEIVED THE DEVICE.

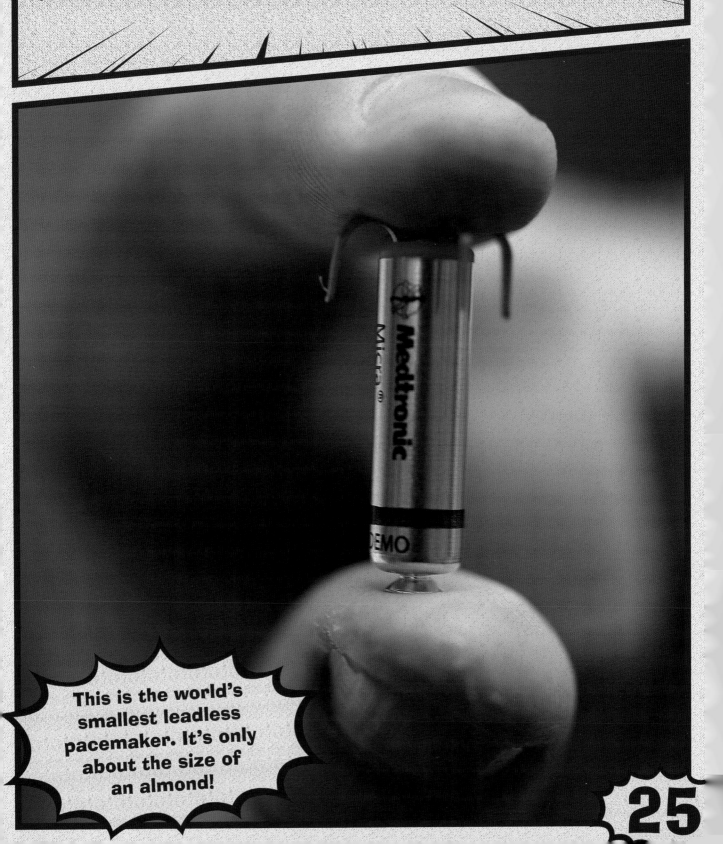

This is the world's smallest leadless pacemaker. It's only about the size of an almond!

ADVANCES IN BIOLOGICAL PACEMAKERS

The artificial pacemaker has developed over the decades, but let's not forget about **biological** pacemakers! These are the cells in your heart that make sure your heart beats in time. Scientists are researching how to use the body's own cells to reset the heart's natural rhythm.

Researchers are starting to understand why pacemaker cells act the way they do. With this information, they hope to "teach" other body cells how to become pacemaker cells. If they can do this, these new cells should be able to set a regular heartbeat. This is exciting research that will hopefully fix problems with the heart's natural pacemaker cells—without the use of a mechanical device.

Using Stem Cells

One way to create new pacemaker cells is by using a person's own **STEM CELLS**. Stem cells are special cells that are able to change into other cell types. Biologists want to be able to encourage stem cells to change into the specific cell type they want, such as pacemaker cells.

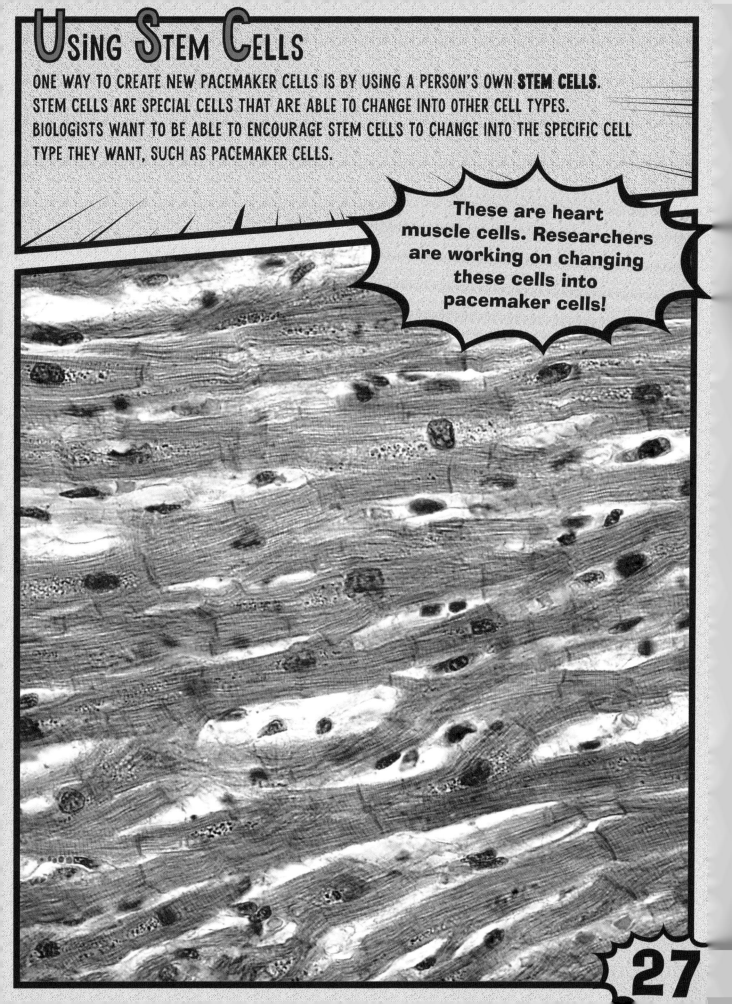

These are heart muscle cells. Researchers are working on changing these cells into pacemaker cells!

A FORTUNATE ACCIDENT

The artificial pacemaker has come a long way, even if its physical journey has only been from outside the body to inside the body. Pacemakers started as a lifesaving tool designed to restart stopped hearts. Since then, the pacemaker has become a standard device many people rely on to live their daily lives.

All around the world, pacemakers help hearts stay in beat. Wilson Greatbatch said that "nine things out of 10 don't work," but for him, the one that worked was an accident! The millions of people who have received an artificial, implantable pacemaker are grateful for that fortunate accident.

John Bell's Pacemaker

AT THE AGE OF 104, JOHN BELL FROM BALTIMORE, MARYLAND, WAS GIVEN A PACEMAKER TO KEEP HIS HEART WORKING WELL. ELEVEN YEARS LATER, IN 1997, HE CAME BACK AFTER THE BATTERY DIED. AT THE AGE OF 115, BELL WAS IN GOOD ENOUGH SHAPE FOR A REPLACEMENT PACEMAKER, SO DOCTORS REPLACED HIS OLD PACEMAKER WITH A NEW ONE!

People have been studying the heart and trying to keep it beating in rhythm for over 100 years. These are some of the major developments.

TIMELINE

1905 — ELECTROCARDIOGRAMS CAPTURE THE BEATING HEART.

1932 — ALBERT HYMAN DEVELOPS A HAND-CRANK MOTOR TO DELIVER ELECTRICAL CURRENTS AND USES THE TERM "ARTIFICIAL PACEMAKER."

1956 — WILSON GREATBATCH ACCIDENTALLY DISCOVERS CERTAIN RESISTORS PRODUCE A HEARTBEAT-LIKE RHYTHM.

1958 — IN MAY, GREATBATCH AND HIS TEAM TEST THEIR PACEMAKERS ON ANIMAL HEARTS.

1958 — IN OCTOBER, RUNE ELMQVIST AND ÅKE SENNING IMPLANT A PACEMAKER IN ARNE LARSSON.

1960 — THE FIRST HUMAN PATIENT RECEIVES A GREATBATCH PACEMAKER.

1972 — LITHIUM-IODINE BATTERIES REPLACE ZINC-MERCURY BATTERIES IN PACEMAKERS.

2000s — THE FIRST BIOLOGICAL PACEMAKER TESTING STARTS.

2009 — THE FIRST PACEMAKER CONNECTED WITH WIRELESS INTERNET IS APPROVED FOR USE.

2016 — THE FIRST LEADLESS PACEMAKER IS APPROVED BY THE US FOOD AND DRUG ADMINISTRATION.

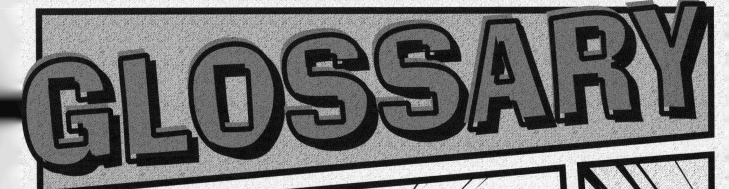

GLOSSARY

biological: relating to life and living things

corrode: to slowly break apart and destroy a metal through a chemical process

engineer: someone who plans and builds machines

implantable: able to be put in a specified place, like someone's body, by means of surgery or an operation

irregular: something that is not regular, or doesn't have a set pattern

laboratory: a place with tools to perform experiments

organ: a body part that does a certain task

reaction: the changes that occur when two chemicals interact with each other

resistor: an electrical device that resists, or slows down current

stem cell: a type of cell in the human body that can change or develop into other types of cells

valve: something that controls the movement of liquids or gases through tubes or vessels

FOR MORE INFORMATION

BOOKS

Biskup, Agnieszka. *Medical Marvels: The Next 100 Years of Medicine*. North Mankato, MN: Capstone Press, 2017.

DK Publishing. *Human Body!* New York, NY: DK Publishing, 2017.

Nagelhout, Ryan. *The Heart and Blood in Your Body*. New York, NY: Britannica Educational Publishing, 2015.

WEBSITES

The Heart

kidshealth.org/en/kids/center/heart-center.html
Watch a quick video to learn how the heart works and discover more about heart problems, getting an EKG, and more.

Pacemakers

www.bhf.org.uk/informationsupport/treatments/pacemakers
Do you want to learn more about the ins and outs of pacemakers? Visit this site to watch videos explaining what a pacemaker is and how it works.

INDEX

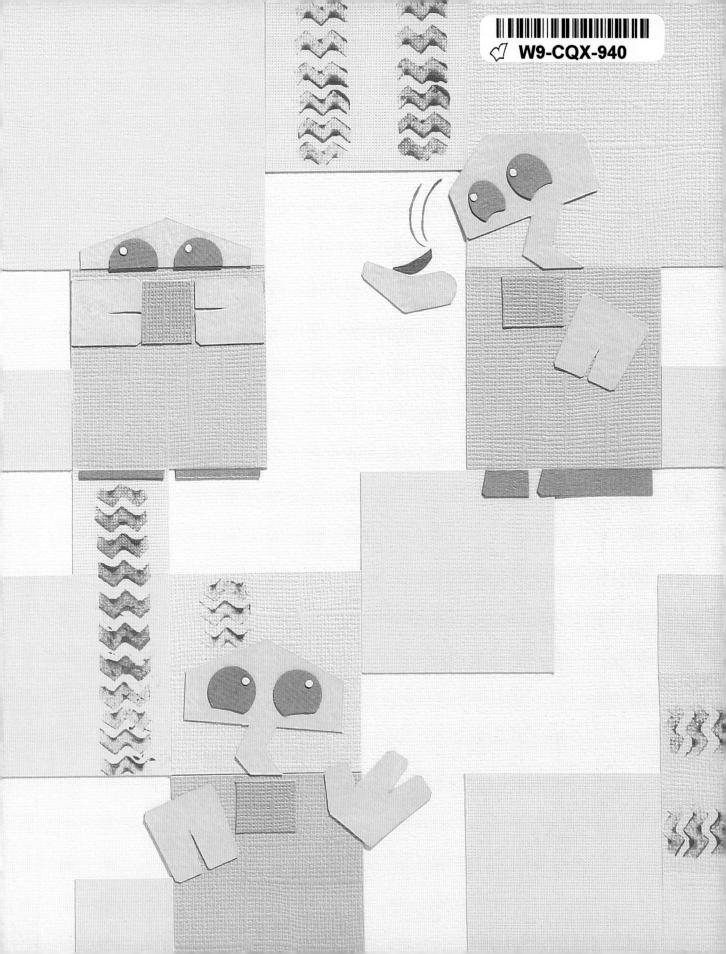

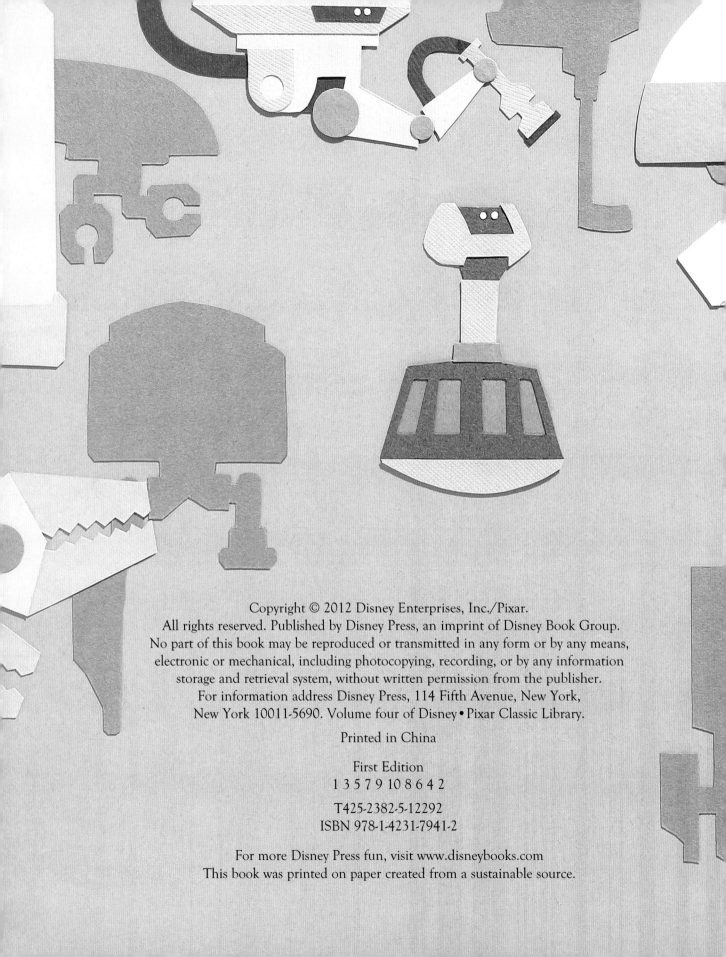

Printed in China

First Edition
1 3 5 7 9 10 8 6 4 2

T425-2382-5-12292
ISBN 978-1-4231-7941-2

For more Disney Press fun, visit www.disneybooks.com
This book was printed on paper created from a sustainable source.

LOTS OF BOTS

By Kiki Thorpe
Illustrated by
Ben Butcher

Disney PRESS
New York

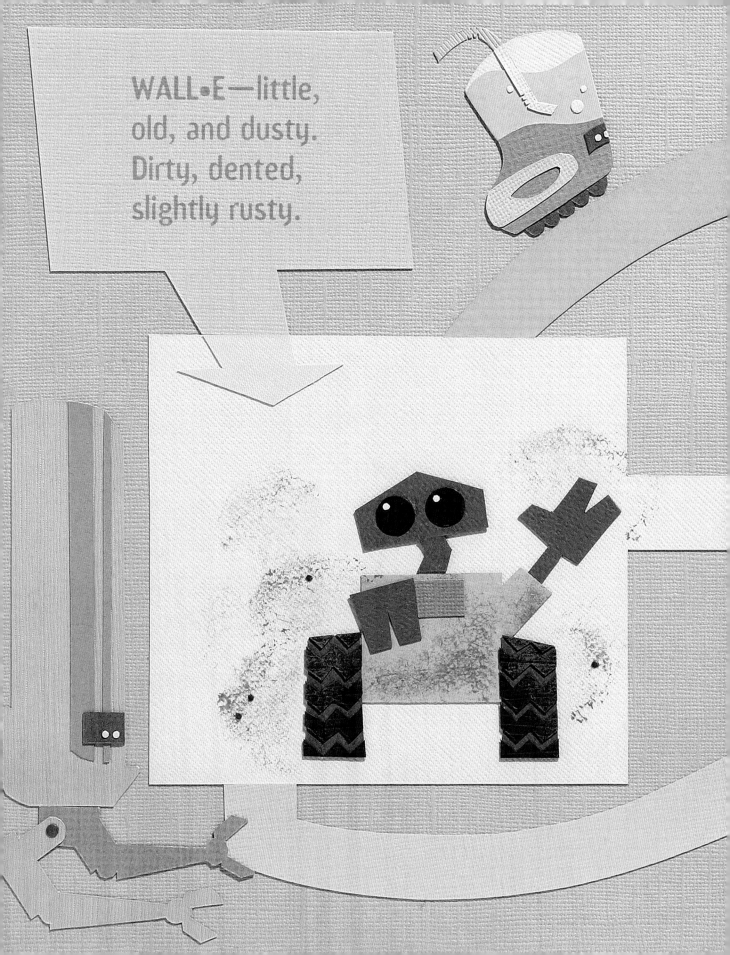

WALL•E—little,
old, and dusty.
Dirty, dented,
slightly rusty.

Scooting.

Sneaking.

HIDING.

Peeking.

Searching ship from end to end,
looking for his special friend.

Line up, robots!

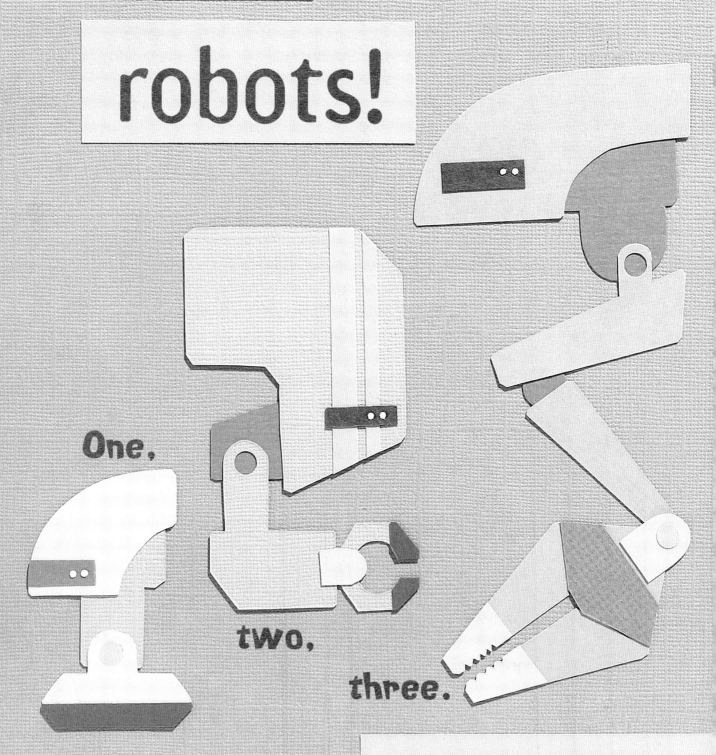

One,

two,

three.

Do the work efficiently.

Look Out!

Robots coming through.

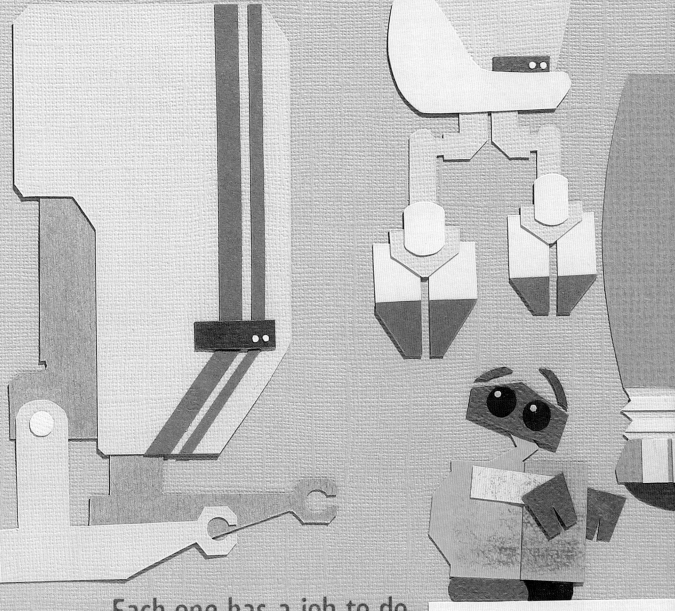

Each one has a job to do.

Scrub-bot **SCOURS.**

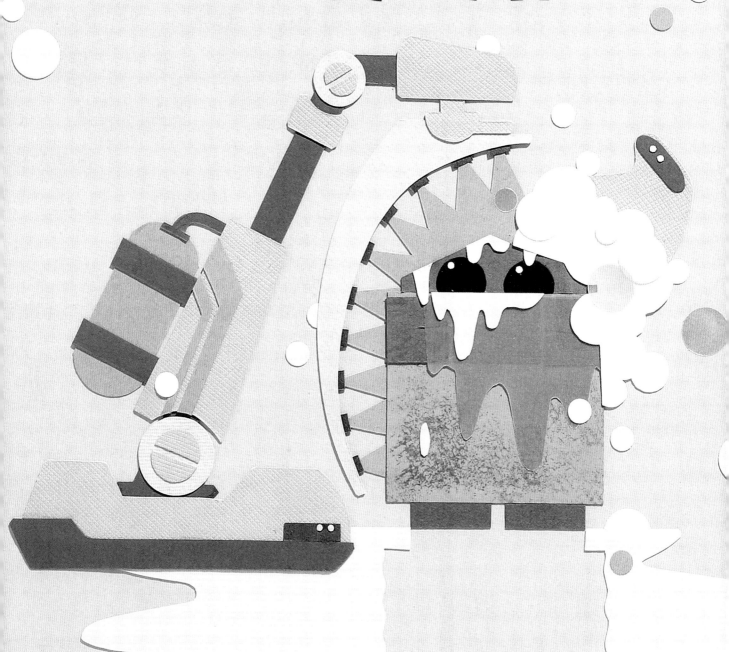

Spray-bot **SHOWERS.**

Paint-bot
coats.

Crane-bot
totes.

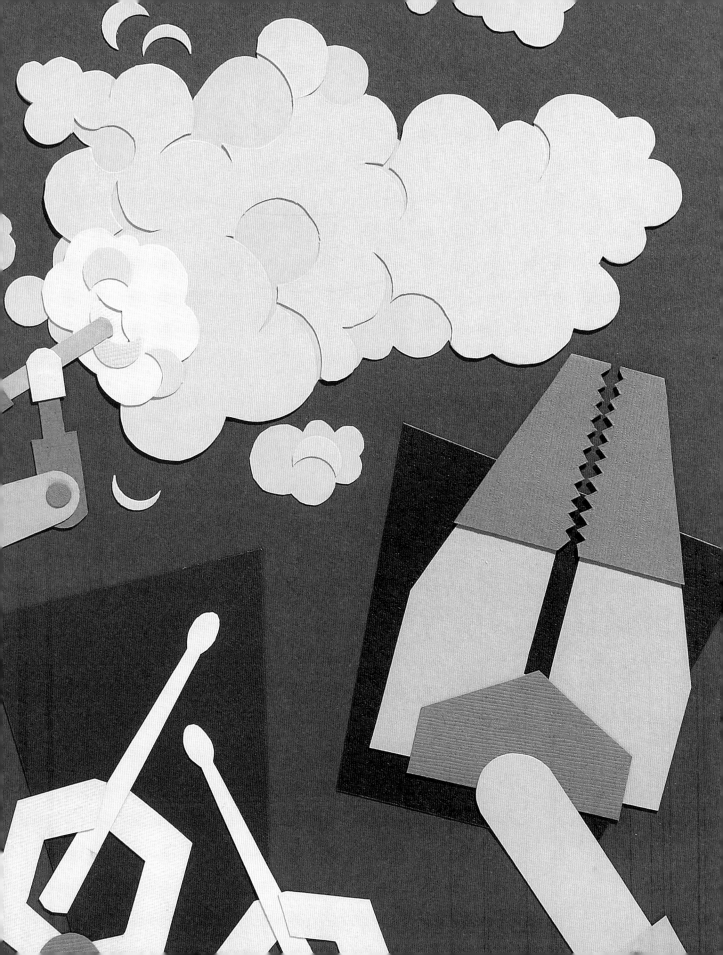

WALL•E sees a bot
for every chore.
But where's the one
he's looking for?

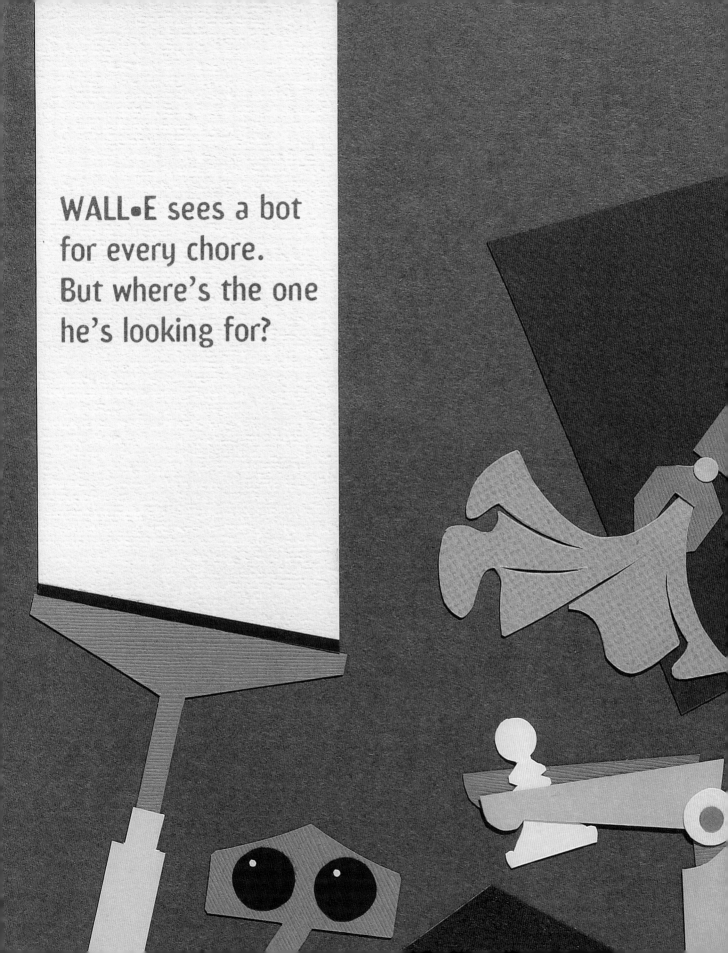

There she is!
At last he sees her.
He can't wait.
He has to reach her.

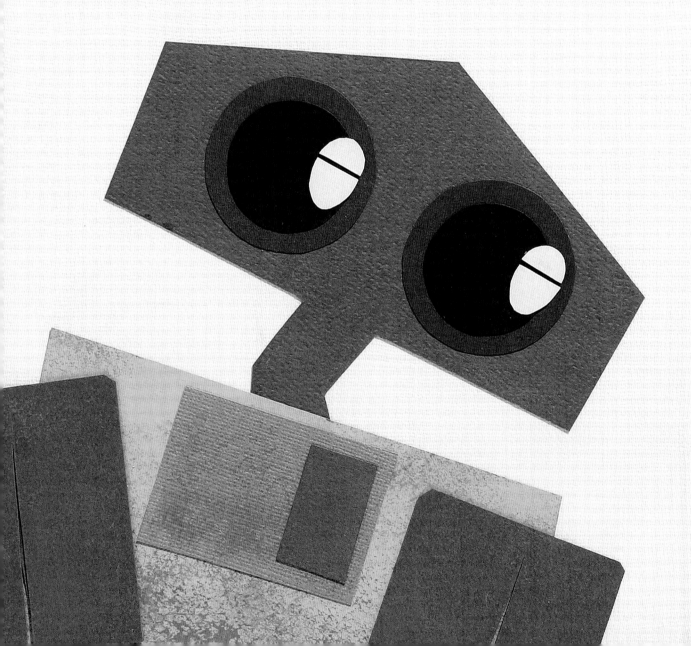

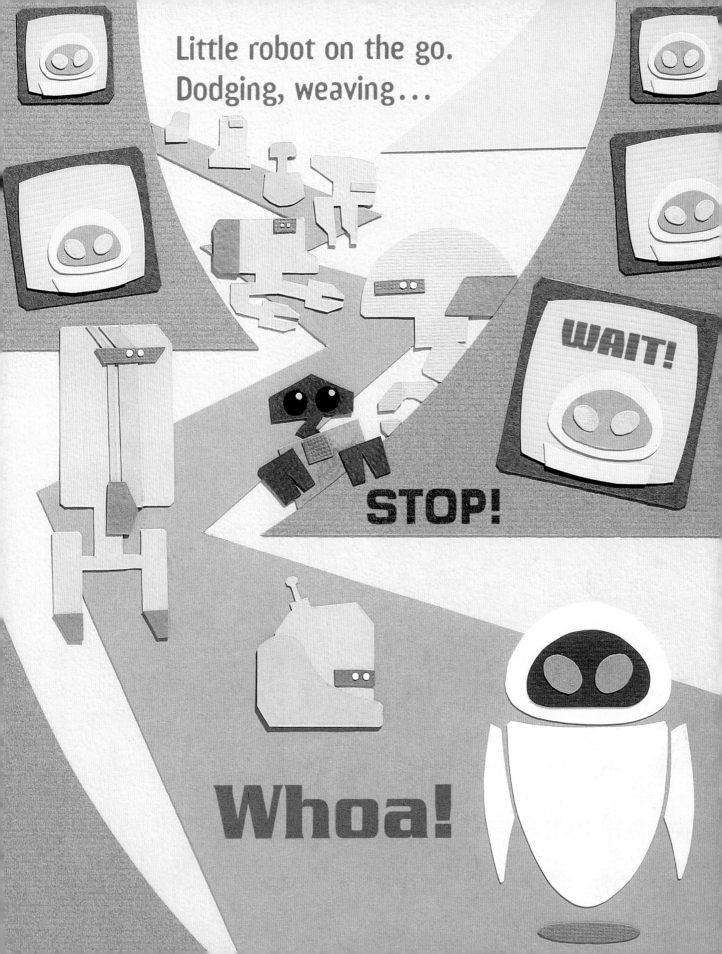

Tractor-bot
crashes.

Forklift-bot
smashes.

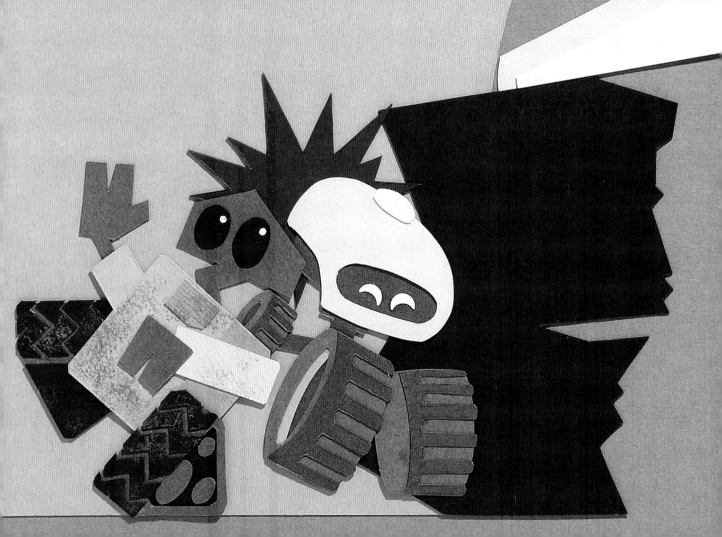

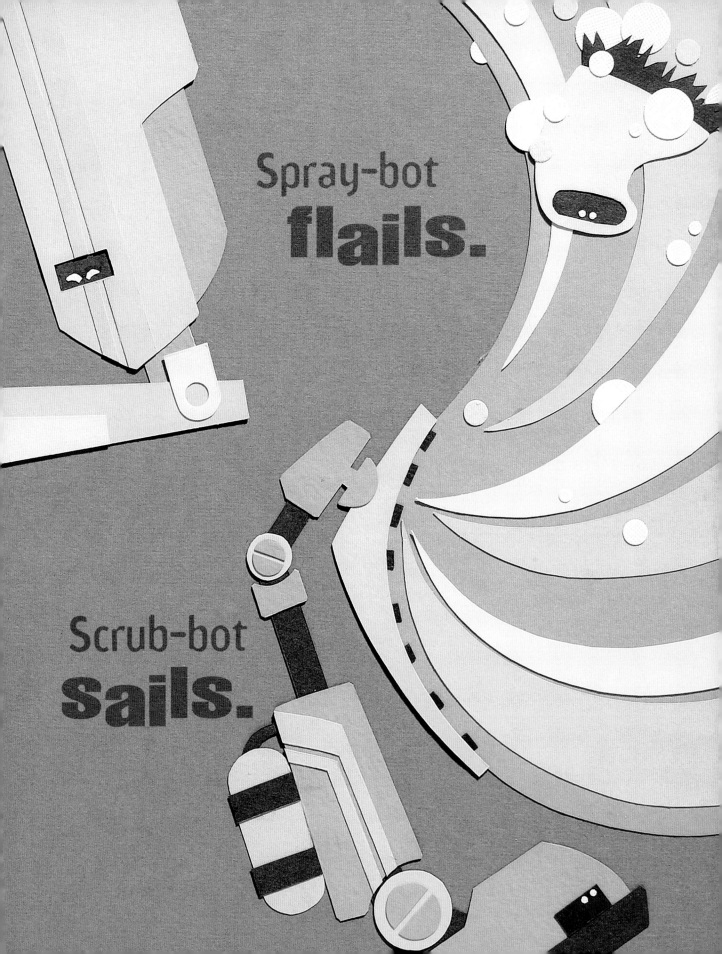

Alarms are **blaring.**

Robots are **staring.**

It's out of **control.**

And here comes the **patrol!**

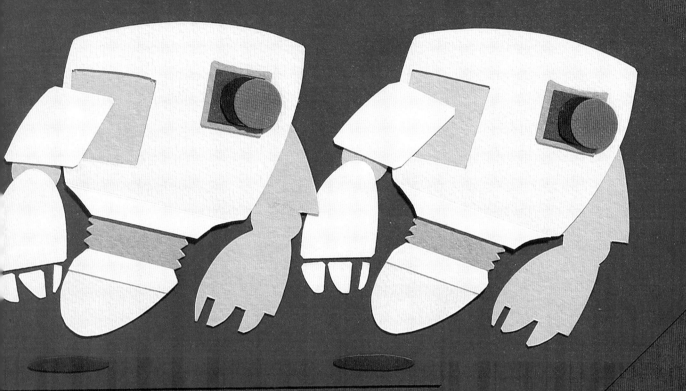

Run **BOTS!**
Race **BOTS!**
Being-chased- **BOTS.**

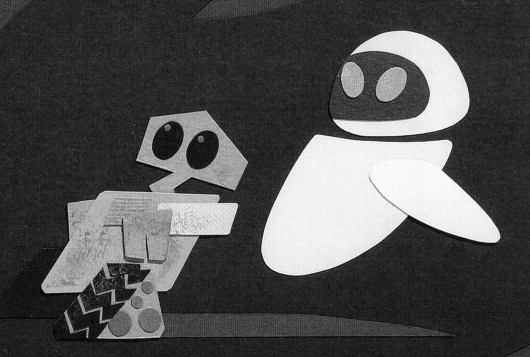

Swerving . . . hopping . . .

oh, NO!

Stopping?

Can't get through!
Only one thing to do.

Music
playing.

Robots
swaying.

Treads start **tapping.**

Clamps are **clapping.**

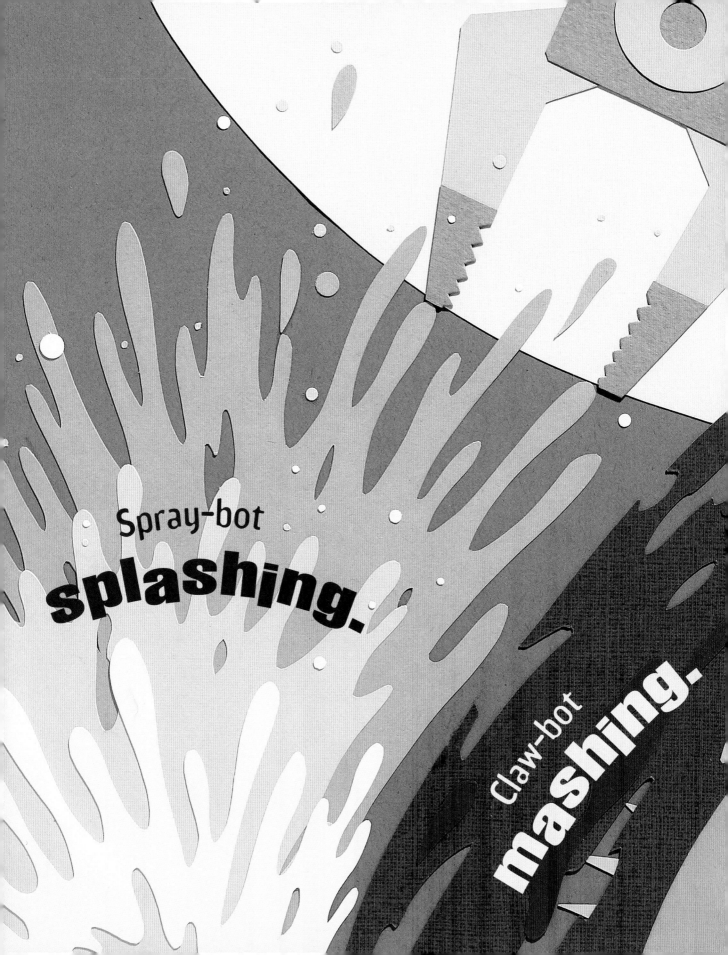

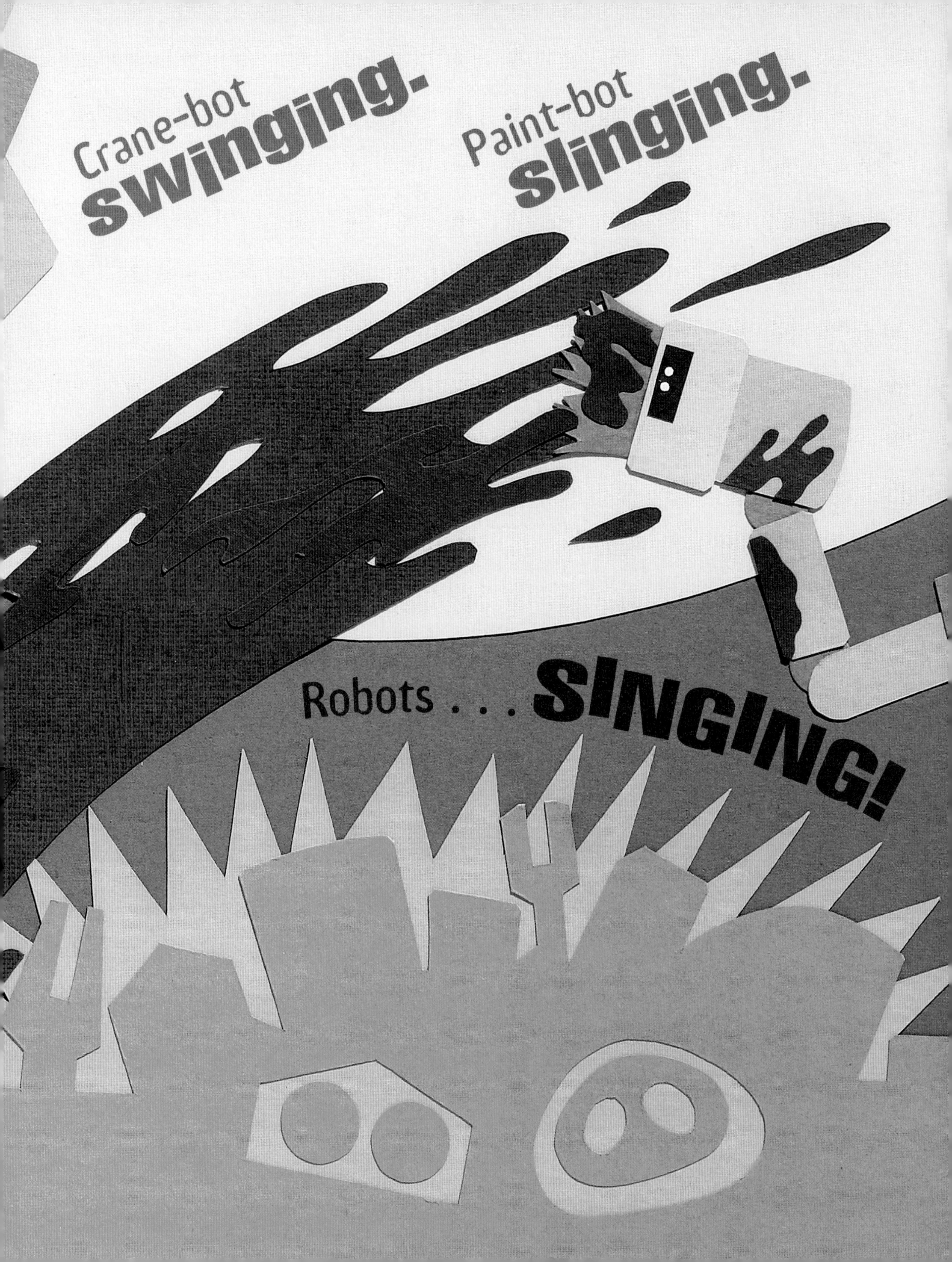

Crane-bot
swinging.

Paint-bot
slinging.

Robots . . . **SINGING!**

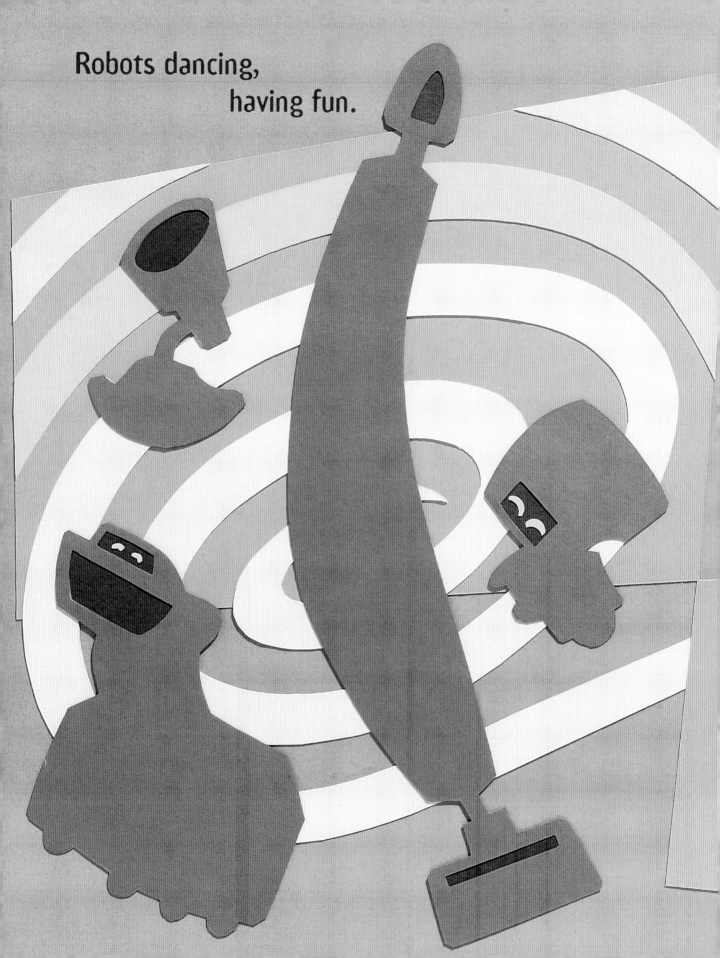

Robots dancing,
        having fun.

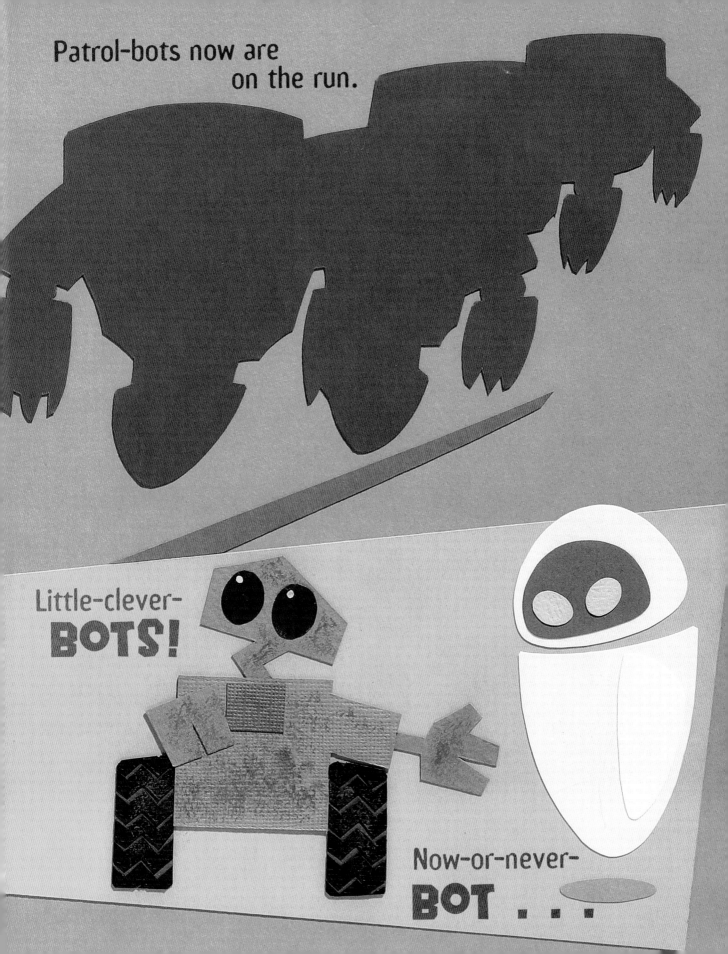

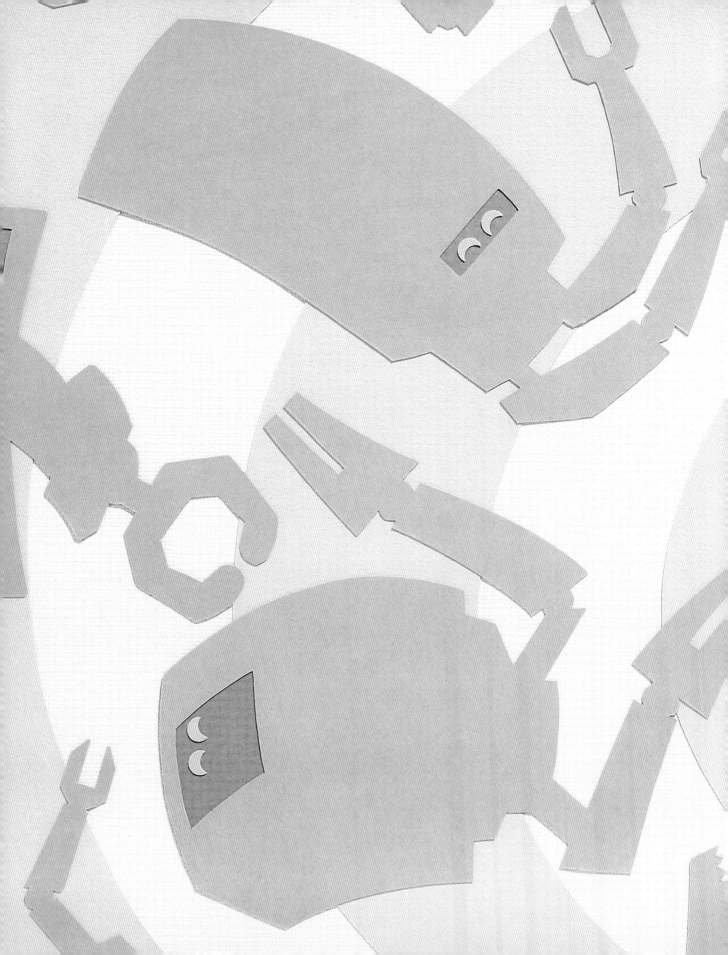

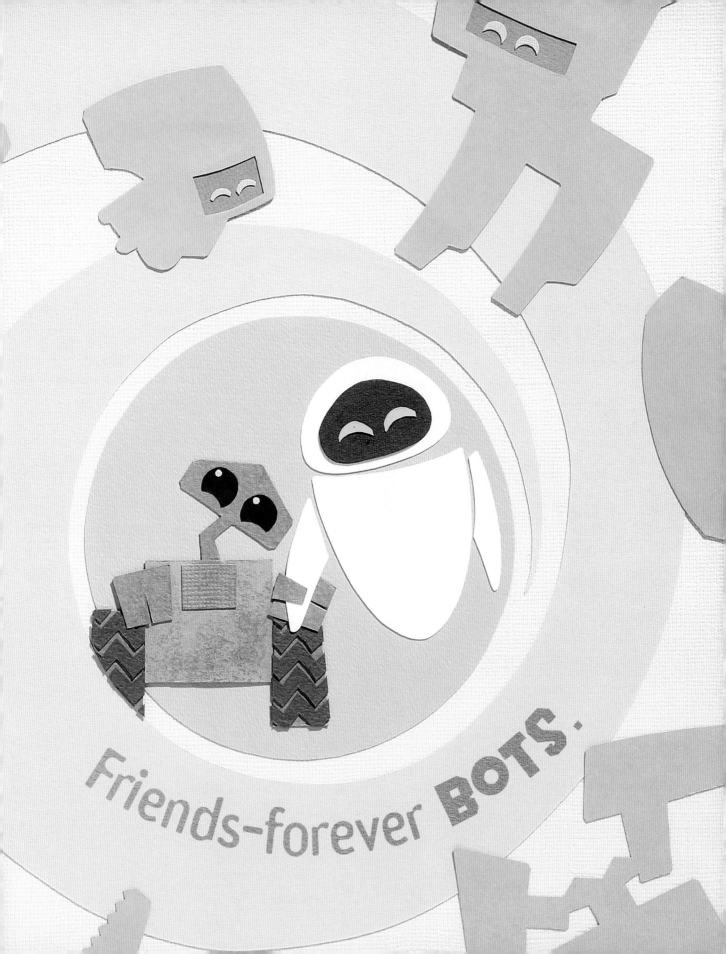

Friends-forever BOTS.

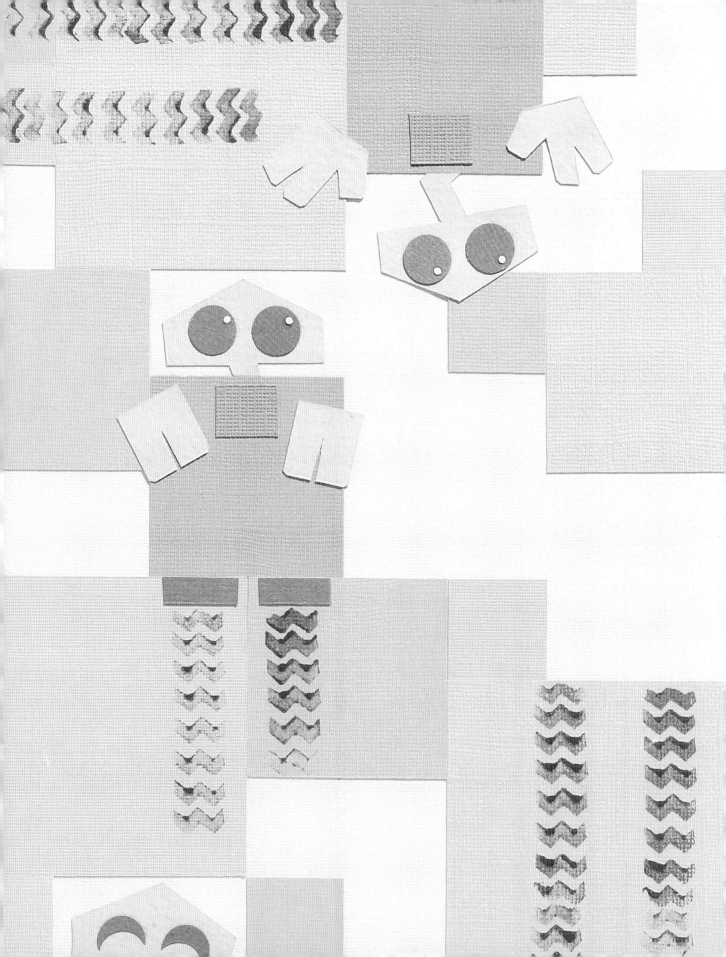